Try It Now! CHICKEN SALADS Volume 2

by Howard Mills

Table of Contents

1. Introduction
2. Peach Grilled Basil Chicken Salad
3. Pickled Persian Chicken Potato Salad
4. Honey Italian Balsamic Chicken Salad
5. Balsamic Blackberry Grilled Chicken Salad with Crispy Fried Goat Cheese
6. Chopped Sriracha Lime Chicken Salad
7. Blue Cheese Chili Chicken Salad

8. Peppered Bacon Cheddar Chicken Salad

9. Bow Tie Mandarin Chicken Salad Pasta

10. Apple Roasted Chicken Salad

11. Grilled Chicken Club Salad with Avocado

12. Kale Chicken Caesar Salad

13. Mexican Chicken and Rice Salad With Black Beans

14. Chopped Apricot and Basil Chicken Salad

15. Shredded Chicken Salad Tostadas

16. Chicken Salad Pita Pockets

17. Garbanzo Bean Pesto Chicken Salad

18. Lemon Yogurt Grilled Chicken Salad

19. Warm Mushroom Chicken-Spinach Salad

20. Pepper Jack Chicken Taco Salad

21. Cashew Chicken Salad

22. Chicken Salad Stuffed Tomatoes and Herbs

23. Warm Potato Bistro Chicken Salad

24. Pistachio Cinnamon Chicken Salad with Greek Yogurt

25. Garlic Sour Cream and Onion Chicken Salad

26. Skinny Honey Chicken Salad

27. Grilled Chicken Bacon and Asparagus Spinach Salad
28. BONUS: 10 More Healthy Foods for Women
29. Conclusion

1. Introduction

Hello and welcome to Part 2 of the healthy eating lifestyle. Thank you for downloading my book. This amazing book contains a compiled list of **25 High Quality chicken salad recipes** that will make your taste buds dance. Each recipe meets **restaurant quality** standards in the comfort of your own kitchen. These Chicken salad recipes will hold your hand and guide you down the path of healthy living.

Hope you all enjoy these fabulous recipes! You also receive a added **BONUS: A list of 10 more healthy foods for women.**

2. Peach Grilled Basil Chicken Salad

Peach Grilled Basil Chicken Salad

Servings 3-4

Ingredients:

*Grilled Basil Chicken

- 1 lb boneless skinless chicken breasts
- 3 Tbsp olive oil, plus more for brushing grill
- 1/3 cup slightly packed chopped fresh basil
- 2 cloves garlic, minced
- 1 Tbsp fresh lemon juice
- Salt and freshly ground black pepper

*Vinaigrette

- 1/3 cup olive oil Coupons

- 3 Tbsp white balsamic vinegar

- 1 Tbsp honey

- 1 tsp dijon mustard

- Salt and freshly ground black pepper

*Salad

- 10 oz Spring Mix lettuce

- 1 lb peaches, sliced (about 3 small)

- 2 ears corn, husked and kernels cut from cob

- 1/2 cup chopped pecans, toasted

- 1/2 small red onion, sliced thin (about 3/4 cup), rinse under water to remove harsh bite

- 4 oz Goat cheese, crumbled

Directions:

*Chicken

1. In a small mixing bowl whisk together olive oil, basil, garlic, and lemon juice and season with salt and pepper (about 1/2 tsp of each). Using the back of a spoon, press basil against sides and bottom of bowl (to help extract flavor from basil). Place chicken in a resealable bag and pound thicker parts of chicken to even thickness with a meat mallet, then pour basil mixture over chicken and evenly distribute basil over chicken. Seal bag while pressing excess air out, rub marinade over chicken and transfer to refrigerator and marinate 2 - 5 hours.

2. Preheat a grill to 425 - 450 degrees over medium high heat. Brush grill grates lightly with olive oil then place chicken on grill. Grill until cooked through, rotating once halfway through cooking, about 4 - 5 minutes per side (chicken should register 165 degrees in center of chicken on an instant read

thermometer). Transfer to a cutting board and let rest 10 minutes then slice into strips or dice into cubes.

*Vinaigrette

1. Whisk together all ingredients until well blended and season with salt and pepper to taste. Store in refrigerator until ready to use, stir again before pouring over salad.

*Salad

1. In a large salad bowl gently toss together lettuce, peaches, corn, pecans, onions, and grilled chicken. Sprinkle goat cheese over top and drizzle with vinaigrette. Serve immediately after adding dressing.

3. Pickled Persian Chicken Potato Salad

Pickled Persian Chicken Potato Salad

Servings 4-5

Ingredients:

- 1 pound russet potatoes
- 3 large eggs
- 3 TBS extra virgin olive oil, divided
- 1 boneless chicken breast
- 1 tsp salt, divided
- 1/4 cup lemon juice
- 3 large dill pickles, diced
- 2 cups frozen peas, thawed
- 1/4 tsp ground black pepper
- 1/4 cup mayonnaise

sliced radishes reduce heat to medium. Continue cooking until potatoes are fork tender. Drain the water and transfer potatoes to a large mixing bowl to cool.

Set eggs in a cold water bath to cool.

While the eggs and potatoes cook, in a small pan over medium-high heat add:

- green onions
- fresh herbs

Directions:

Wash and peel:

- 1 pound russet potatoes

Cut the potatoes in quarters, place in a large saucepan and cover with water.

*Add with the potatoes

- 3 large eggs

- 1 TBS extra virgin olive oil

- 1 boneless chicken breast

Season chicken breast with:

- 1/4 tsp salt

Cook until the chicken breast is browned, then flip over and cook other side of chicken breast. Season second chicken side with:

- 1/4 tsp salt

Reduce heat to low and add:

- 2 TBS lemon juice

Cover pan and continue cooking until chicken is cooked thoroughly and juices run clear, about 15 minutes.

Remove chicken from heat and cool.

When potatoes are cool to touch, coarsely cut into 1/2-inch pieces in the mixing bowl.

Peel the cooked eggs, dice and add to the potatoes.

Dice the cooled chicken breast and add to the mix.

*Add to the potato mix:

- 3 large dill pickles, diced
- 2 cups frozen peas, thawed
- 1/4 tsp ground black pepper
- 1/2 tsp salt

Mix the ingredients together.

Stir in until smooth:

- 1/4 cup mayonnaise
- 2 TBS lemon juice
- 2 TBS extra virgin olive oil

Cover and refrigerate salad until ready to serve.

When ready to serve, transfer salad to a serving plate and smooth into a round mound.

Garnish as you please with:

- sliced radishes
- green onions
- fresh herbs

Serve.

4. Honey Italian Balsamic Chicken Salad

Honey Italian Balsamic Chicken Salad

Ingredients:

*Chicken

- 2 chicken breasts boneless and skinless
- 2 cloves of garlic minced
- 2 teaspoons of mustard
- 2 teaspoons of honey
- ¼ teaspoon of salt
- ½ teaspoon pepper
- Pinch of chili flakes optional
- ¼ cup of balsamic vinegar

- 1 teaspoon of honey or brown sugar

- 1 cup of chicken stock

*Salad

- 1 cup of sliced roast beets

- ½ cup of blackberries

- 2 avocados sliced

- 1 res onion sliced

- 3 cups of greens (spinach, kale , spring mix)

- ¼ cup of Bocconcini

- For the dressing;

- 2 tablespoons of minced shallots

- 1 tablespoon of fresh rosemary leaves minced

- 2 tablespoons of fresh blackberries minced

- 1 teaspoon of honey

- 1 tablespoon of mustard

- ⅛ teaspoon of salt

- ¼ cup of balsamic vinegar

- ½ cup of olive oil

Directions:

1. Start off with the chicken. Mix all ingredients together and preheat a grill pan on medium high heat.

2. Add the chicken reserving any extra balsamic mixture, and grill 5 min, on each side. Then add the reserved balsamic marinade with the stock, cover the chicken and let it cook through for 5 min, on medium heat.

3. In the meantime arrange the salad bowl.

4. Prepare the dressing in a small food container. Add all ingredients, place the lid on and shake the container until the dressing comes together.

5. Slice the chicken and arrange it over the salad, then pour about 2 tablespoons of the dressing evenly over the salad.

6. Serve.

5. Balsamic Blackberry Grilled Chicken Salad with Crispy Fried Goat Cheese

Balsamic Blackberry Grilled Chicken Salad with Crispy Fried Goat Cheese

Servings: 4

Ingredients:

*Dressing

- 1/2 cup blackberries
- 2 tablespoons white balsamic vinegar
- 2 tablespoons extra virgin olive oil
- 2 tablespoons honey
- 2 teaspoons Dijon mustard
- 1 teaspoon tamari or soy sauce

- 1 large clove garlic, minced

- salt and pepper to taste

*Fried Goat Cheese

- 8 ounces goat cheese, either sliced into 1/4 inch thick discs or formed into small balls

- 1/4 cup flour

- 1 large egg, lightly beaten

- 1 cup panko breadcrumbs (or breadcrumbs)

*Salad

- 1/2 pound chicken breasts

- 6 cups lettuce

- 1 cup blackberries

- 1 avocado, sliced

- 1/4 cup red onion, sliced

- 1/4 cup walnuts (or pistachios or almonds)

Directions:

*Dressing

1. Mix everything well.

*Goat Cheese

1. Dredge the goat cheese slices/balls in the flour and coat in egg followed by breadcrumbs and fry in oil over medium heat until lightly golden brown before setting aside on paper towels to drain.

*Salad

1. Marinate the chicken in half of the vinaigrette for 30 minutes to over night before grilling over medium-high heat until cooked and slightly charred, about 2-5 minutes per side, and setting aside to cool and slice.

2. Assemble the salad and serve.

6. Chopped Sriracha Lime Chicken Salad

Chopped Sriracha Lime Chicken Salad

Servings 2-3

Ingredients:

*Sriracha Lime Chicken

- 2 organic chicken breasts
- 3 tablespoons sriracha
- 1 lime, juiced
- 1/4 teaspoon fine sea salt
- 1/4 teaspoon freshly ground pepper

*Salad

- 4 cups lettuce, chopped
- 8 pineapple slices, using pineapple corer
- 1 cup organic grape tomatoes
- 1/3 cup red onion, finely chopped
- 1 avocado, cubed

*Lime Vinaigrette

- 1/3 cup light olive oil
- 1/4 cup apple cider vinegar
- 2 limes, juiced
- 2 tsp raw honey
- Dash fine sea salt

Directions:

1. Heat the grill to medium heat.

2. Season chicken with salt and pepper. In a bowl or marinade dish, combine sriracha and lime.

3. Add chicken and let marinade in the fridge for at least 20 minutes, the longer the better.

4. Once ready to cook, add chicken to the greased grill.

5. Cut pineapple using pineapple corer and add to grill, grill for 3-4 minutes on each side.

6. While they are grilling, chop lettuce, then chop avocado, tomato, and red onion and add to serving dish.

7. Whisk together dressing, taste, and adjust seasoning as desired place in fridge until ready to use.

8. Once chicken is done cooking, assemble the salad, toss with dressing and serve.

7. Blue Cheese Chili Chicken Salad

Blue Cheese Chili Chicken Salad

Servings 4

Ingredients:

- 12 chicken tenderloins (1-1/4 to 1-1/2 lbs)

- 1 large egg, lightly beaten

- 1 tablespoon milk

- 1-1/4 cups dry breadcrumbs

- 1 teaspoon salt

- Freshly ground black pepper

- Vegetable oil

- 3 tablespoons butter

- 1/3 cup sweet Thai chili sauce

- 12 ounces mixed greens (romaine, red leaf lettuce, baby spinach, etc.)
- 2 medium ripe or 12 Campari tomatoes, cut into wedges
- 1/2 English cucumber, peeled and sliced
- 1/2 medium red bell pepper, seeded and cut into this strips

*Blue Cheese Ranch Dressing

- 1/3 cup buttermilk
- 1/3 cup mayonnaise
- 1 tablespoon white wine vinegar
- 1/4 cup vegetable oil
- 1 large clove garlic, very finely chopped
- Salt and freshly ground black pepper
- 1/3 cup crumbled blue cheese (or more to taste)

Directions:

1. Prepare the dressing by whisking the buttermilk, mayonnaise, vinegar, oil and garlic together in a small bowl. Season to taste with salt and pepper and stir in the blue cheese.

2. Trim any small white tendons from the chicken tenderloins and set aside. In a shallow dish like a pie plate, whisk the egg and milk together until well blended. Combine the breadcrumbs, salt and pepper and spread on a dinner plate or sheet of wax paper.

3. Dip each piece of chicken first in the egg, then in the crumb mixture, pressing lightly to be sure the crumbs adhere well.

4. Add about 1/8-inch of vegetable oil to a large skillet and heat over medium-high heat. Add the tenderloins in a single layer and cook until the crumb coating is golden brown and their interior is no longer pink, 2 to 3 minutes per side.

5. Transfer the cooked tenderloins to a paper towel-lined plate to drain and wipe the excess oil from the pan.

6. Return the pan to the stove over medium heat and add the butter and sweet Thai chili sauce. Once the butter has melted, combine well, then return the chicken to the pan.

7. Carefully turn the tenderloins several times to coat them with chili sauce mixture. Remove the pan from the heat and set aside.

8. To serve, divide the greens between 4 plates and arrange the cucumber, red bell pepper and tomatoes around the edges. Place 3 pieces of chicken in the center of each plate and spoon about 2 tablespoons of dressing over the salad.

8. Peppered Bacon Cheddar Chicken Salad

Peppered Bacon Cheddar Chicken Salad

Servings 2-3

Ingredients:

- 3 large chicken breasts
- 4-6 strips peppered bacon, cooked and crumbled
- 1 packet powdered chicken flavored bouillon
- Salt & pepper
- 1 ½ cup (5 oz.) shredded cheddar cheese
- ½ cup mayonnaise
- ½ cup sour cream
- 2 tablespoons chopped chives
- Crackers, bread, or assorted veggies for dipping

Direction:

1. Boil chicken in water with 1 packet of the bouillon. Boil for about 10 minutes until its all cooked through, then move to the bowl of your mixer. Using the whisk attachment, turn mixer on to shred chicken (or do it by hand or with some forks).

2. In a large bowl, mix mayonnaise and sour cream add chicken, cheese, crumbled bacon and most of the chives. Season with salt and pepper. Move to your serving dish and top with chives.

3. Refrigerate until ready to serve.

9. Bow Tie Mandarin Chicken Salad Pasta

Bow Tie Mandarin Chicken Salad Pasta

Servings 4-5

Ingredients:

- 1 teaspoon finely chopped, peeled fresh ginger
- 1/3 cup rice vinegar
- 1/4 cup orange juice
- 1/4 cup vegetable oil
- 1 teaspoon toasted sesame oil
- 1 (1 ounce) package dry onion soup mix
- 2 teaspoons white sugar
- 1 clove garlic, pressed
- 1 (8 ounce) package bow tie (farfalle) pasta

*Barilla Pasta

- 1/2 cucumber - scored, halved lengthwise, seeded, and sliced

- 1/2 cup diced red bell pepper

- 1/2 cup coarsely chopped red onion

- 2 diced Roma tomatoes

- 1 carrot, shredded

- 1 (6 ounce) bag fresh spinach

- 1 (11 ounce) can mandarin orange segments, drained

- 2 cups diced cooked chicken

- 1/2 cup sliced almonds, toasted

Directions:

1. To make the dressing, whisk together the ginger root, rice vinegar, orange juice, vegetable oil, sesame oil, soup mix, sugar, and garlic until well blended. Cover, and refrigerate until needed.

2. Bring a large pot of lightly salted water to a boil. Add the bow tie pasta and cook for 8 to 10 minutes. Drain, and rinse under cold water. Place pasta in a large bowl.

3. To make the salad, toss the cucumber, bell pepper, onion, tomatoes, carrot, spinach, mandarin oranges, chicken, and almonds with the pasta. Pour the dressing over the salad mixture, and toss again to coat evenly. Serve immediately.

10. Apple Roasted Chicken Salad

Apple Roasted Chicken Salad

Servings 3

Ingredients:

- 1 cup pecan halves (about 3 ounces), broken in half lengthwise

- 1 whole roasted chicken (about 3 pounds), skin removed

- 8 scallions, white and light-green parts only, trimmed and thinly sliced

- 2 stalks celery, strings removed and thinly sliced

- 8 ounces lady apples (about 4), or Fuji apples (about 2 medium), cored and sliced into bite-size pieces

- 5 tablespoons golden or dark raisins

- 1 tablespoon coarsely chopped fresh oregano leaves

- Coarse salt and freshly ground pepper

- Sour Cream Dressing

Directions:

1. Preheat oven to 350 degrees. Spread pecans in a single layer on a rimmed baking sheet. Toast in oven until fragrant, stirring occasionally, about 10 minutes. Remove from pan; let cool completely.

2. Pull chicken from the bone; discard bones, and cut meat into 3/4-inch pieces. Transfer to a medium bowl; add scallions, celery, apples, raisins, and oregano. Season with salt and pepper. Add dressing; toss to combine. Chill, covered, until ready to serve.

11. Grilled Chicken Club Salad with Avocado

Grilled Chicken Club Salad with Avocado

Servings 3

Ingredients:

*Grilled Chicken

- 1 tbsp. smoked paprika
- 1 tsp. garlic powder
- 1 tsp. onion powder
- 1/2 tsp. sea salt
- several grinds pepper
- 16 ounces chicken breast, trimmed of fat
- Creamy Avocado Dressing
- 1 avocado, skin and pit removed

- 1/4 cup greek yogurt

- 1 tbsp. white wine vinegar

- 1 shallot, chopped

- salt and pepper

- 1/4 cup buttermilk

*Salad

- Croutons

- 4 slices bacon, fried crisp, and crumbled

- 6 cups leafy greens

- 4 ounces tiny tomatoes, halved lengthwise

- 1 avocado, cubed

- grilled chicken, cubed

Directions:

1. Preheat grill. Combine rub ingredients for grilled chicken. Rub spice mix into the chicken breast. Grill chicken.

2. When cool, cube, and set aside.

3. Preheat oven to 400 degrees. Cube bread. Toss with a drizzle of olive oil. Spread on a baking sheet - a single layer. Bake until golden brown - about 10 minutes. Set aside.

4. Make dressing. Combine all ingredients in blender. Pulse until smooth. Check for seasoning and consistency. If the mixture is too thick, add additional buttermilk. Dressing should be thick and creamy, not runny. Set aside.

5. To a large salad bowl, add greens. Toss with a conservative amount of dressing. Add crumbled bacon, tomatoes, cubed avocado, cubed grilled chicken, and croutons. Serve remaining dressing on the side.

12. Kale Chicken Caesar Salad

Kale Chicken Caesar Salad

Servings 4

Ingredients:

- 2 tablespoons extra-virgin olive oil

- 3 ounces whole-wheat bread, torn into 1-inch pieces (about 2 cups)

- 2/3 cup low-fat buttermilk

- 1/4 cup grated Parmesan (about 1 ounce)

- 2 tablespoons reduced-fat sour cream

- 1 lemon, 1/2 juiced (1 tablespoon juice) and 1/2 cut into 4 wedges

- 1 small clove garlic, grated

- Kosher salt and freshly ground black pepper

- 12 ounces cooked shredded chicken

- 1 large bunch kale (about 1 pound), stems discarded, leaves thinly sliced

Directions:

1. Heat 1 tablespoon oil in a medium nonstick skillet set over medium heat. Add the bread pieces and cook, stirring, until lightly golden and a bit crisp, about 5 minutes. Remove from the heat and set aside to cool in the skillet. They will continue to crisp up as they cool.

2. Whisk together the buttermilk, 2 tablespoons of the Parmesan, the sour cream, remaining 1 tablespoon olive oil, the lemon juice and garlic in a small bowl and until smooth. Season with pepper and 1/4 teaspoon salt.

3. Toss together the chicken, kale and croutons with the dressing in a large bowl until well coated. Divide among 4 plates, sprinkle

evenly with the remaining 2 tablespoons Parmesan and serve with a lemon wedge.

13. Mexican Chicken and Rice Salad With Black Beans

Mexican Chicken and Rice Salad With Black Beans

Servings 2

Ingredients:

- 1 tbsp olive oil
- 2 chicken breasts, cut into small pieces
- 1½ cups cooked rice, I used basmati
- 1 green bell pepper, chopped
- 1 cup cherry tomatoes, chopped
- 1 cup frozen corn
- 1 cup black beans
- 6 green onions, chopped

- 1 cup queso duro, shredded
- ½ cup cilantro, chopped
- 3 tbsp taco seasoning
- juice from 1 lemon
- juice from 1 lime
- 2 tbsp olive oil
- salt and pepper to taste
- 1 avocado (optional)

Directions:

1. Heat olive oil in a non stick skillet over medium high heat. Season the chicken with the taco seasoning, add more if you want it spicier, and add chicken to skillet. Cook chicken for about 10 minutes until cooked through and starts to slightly brown. Remove chicken from skillet.

2. To the same skillet add the corn and cook over high heat just until it starts to char a little bit, no more than 2 minutes.

3. Add all ingredients to a large bowl, season with salt and pepper and toss.

4. Serve.

14. Chopped Apricot and Basil Chicken Salad

Chopped Apricot and Basil Chicken Salad

Servings 1-2

Ingredients:

- 1/3 cup mayonnaise

- 1/2 cup Greek yogurt

- 1 garlic clove, minced

- 1/2 teaspoon smoked paprika

- 2 tablespoons champagne or white wine vinegar

- 3 cups shredded cooked chicken

- 1/4 cup blanched slivered almonds, toasted

- 1/2 cup finely diced white onion or shallot

- 1 cup diced celery, with leaves if possible

- 1/2 cup dried apricots, chopped

- 1/3 cup packed fresh basil leaves, cut into thin strips

- 1 tablespoon poppy seeds

- Coarse salt and freshly ground pepper

- Crackers or sandwich bread, for serving

Directions:

1. Whisk together the mayonnaise, yogurt, garlic, paprika and vinegar in a large bowl. Fold in the chicken, almonds, onion, celery, apricots, basil and poppy seeds. Season with salt and pepper to taste.

2. Cover and refrigerate for at least 2 hours to allow the flavors to meld, then serve with your favorite crackers or sandwich bread.

15. Shredded Chicken Salad Tostadas

Shredded Chicken Salad Tostadas

Servings 4-5

Ingredients:

- 2 chicken breasts
- 1 tsp kosher salt
- 1 tsp black pepper
- 1 red pepper diced
- 1/4 cup red onion diced
- 2 cups corn or 1 can
- 2 cups black beans
- 1/2 bunch cilantro rinsed and minced
- 1/2 cup mayonnaise
- 15 tostadas

- 1 avocado optional for topping

Directions:

1. Add 2 chicken breasts to your crock pot with 4 cups of water. Sprinkle the salt and pepper over the top and allow it to cook for the desired amount of time. You can also boil the chicken on the stove top. Boil it on high for 25 minutes.

2. Once the chicken has cooked, remove it from the crock pot and leave it on a plate to rest for 15 minutes. This will make sure the moisture will stay inside the meat and not dry out. Meanwhile dice the red pepper, onions, cilantro. Put it in a large bowl with the corn and the beans. Mix them together.

3. Shred the chicken breasts. Add the shredded chicken to the bowl of vegetables.

4. Add the 1/2 cup of mayonnaise and mix.

5. Top each tostada with the chicken salad mixture. Add avocado if desired.

6. Serve.

16. Chicken Salad Pita Pockets

Chicken Salad Pita Pockets

Servings 6

Ingredients:

- 2 cups cubed cooked chicken

- 1-1/2 cups seedless red grapes, halved

- 1 cup chopped cucumber

- 3/4 cup sliced almonds

- 3/4 cup shredded part-skim mozzarella cheese

- 1/2 cup poppy seed salad dressing

- 6 pita pocket halves

- Leaf lettuce, optional

Directions:

1. In a large bowl, combine the chicken, grapes, cucumber, almonds and mozzarella cheese. Drizzle with dressing and toss to coat. Line pita breads with lettuce if desired; fill with chicken salad and serve.

17. Garbanzo Bean Pesto Chicken Salad

Garbanzo Bean Pesto Chicken Salad

Servings 2-3

Ingredients:

- 1 lb skinless, boneless chicken breasts, cooked and shredded

- 2 medium sized cucumbers (4 Persian cucumbers), sliced

- 4 cups salad greens

- 1 cup garbanzo beans, drained and rinsed

- 4 green onions, sliced

- Juice of 1 lemon

- 2 cups whole, fresh basil leaves

- 2 cloves garlic, chopped

- 1/4 cup grated Parmesan cheese

- 1 tbsp olive oil

- 2 tbsp water

- Salt and pepper to taste

Directions:

1. Make pesto sauce by adding the basil leaves, garlic, Parmesan cheese, olive oil, water, and salt & pepper to a food processor and pulse to combine.

2. In a large bowl, combine lettuce, cucumbers, garbanzo beans, chicken and green onions. Drizzle in the basil pesto dressing, and toss to coat.

3. Divide evenly into 4 bowls, squeeze lemon juice over each one, season with addition salt and pepper, and serve.

18. Lemon Yogurt Grilled Chicken Salad

Lemon Yogurt Grilled Chicken Salad

Servings 3-4

Ingredients:

*Chicken

- 1/3 cup plain Greek yogurt
- 1 tbsp lemon pepper seasoning
- 1/4 tsp garlic powder
- 3 tbsp lemon juice
- 1 tbsp olive oil
- 2 lbs thin-sliced boneless skinless chicken breasts
- Salt, as desired

*Dressing

- 3 tbsp lemon juice

- 1/2 cup plain Greek yogurt

- 3 tbsp olive oil

- 1/2 clove garlic, minced

- 1/4 tsp kosher salt

- Freshly cracked black pepper, to taste

*Salad

- 3 medium zucchini, halved

- Olive oil, for brushing

- Salt and pepper, as desired

- Spinach, or other salad

Directions:

1. Place chicken, yogurt, lemon pepper seasoning, garlic powder, lemon juice, and olive oil into a gallon-sized plastic storage bag. Shake to coat evenly. Marinate chicken in refrigerator for at least 4 hours.

2. Remove chicken from marinade and sprinkle with salt, as desired.

3. Brush zucchini halves lightly with olive oil and season with salt and pepper, as desired.

4. Over grill heated to medium-high, grill chicken for 3-4 minutes each side, or until internal temperature reaches 165°F.

5. Grill zucchini for 2-3 minutes per side.

6. Assemble dressing by whisking together lemon juice, yogurt, olive oil, garlic, salt and pepper.

7. Top spinach with chicken, zucchini, and dressing.

8. Serve.

19. Warm Mushroom Chicken-Spinach Salad

Warm Mushroom Chicken-Spinach Salad

Servings 1-2

Ingredients:

- 3 tbsp. olive oil
- 1 large red onion
- ½ tsp. salt
- ¼ tsp. coarsely ground pepper
- 2 package assorted sliced wild mushrooms
- ⅓ c. cider vinegar
- 1 tbsp. sugar
- 2 bag baby spinach
- 2 c. rotisserie chicken meat

Directions:

1. In nonstick 12-inch skillet, heat 1 tablespoon oil over medium-high heat until hot. Add onion, salt, and pepper, and cook 10 minutes or until onion is tender and golden, stirring occasionally. Add mushrooms and cook 5 minutes or until mushrooms are browned and liquid evaporates.

2. Stir vinegar, sugar, and remaining 2 tablespoons oil into mushroom mixture. Heat to boiling; boil 30 seconds, stirring.

3. In large serving bowl, toss spinach and chicken with warm dressing until salad is evenly coated. Serve immediately.

20. Pepper Jack Chicken Taco Salad

Pepper Jack Chicken Taco Salad

Servings 2-3

Ingredients:

*Dressing

- 3/4 cups Ranch Dressing
- 1/4 cup Salsa
- 3 Tablespoons Finely Minced Cilantro

*Chicken

- 2 whole Boneless, Skinless Chicken Breasts

- 2 Tablespoons Seasoning of taco Seasoning,

- 1/4 cup Vegetable Oil

- 2 Tablespoons of Butter

*Salad

- 1 head Green Leaf Lettuce Shredded Thin

- 3 whole Roma Tomatoes, Diced

- 1/2 cup Grated Pepper Jack Cheese

- 2 ears Corn, Shucked

- 2 whole Avocados, Diced

- 3 whole Green Onions, Sliced

- 1/2 cup Cilantro Leaves

- Tortilla Chips Of Your Choice, Crushed Slightly

Directions:

1. First, make the dressing by combining all the ingredients in a bowl and stirring together. Cover and refrigerate.

2. Next, make the chicken: Generously season both sides of the breasts. Heat the oil and butter in a large skillet over medium-high heat. Cook the chicken on both sides until deep golden brown on the outside and done in the middle, about 4 minutes per side. Remove and set aside to cool for 10 minutes, then cut it into cubes.

3. Place the ears of corn in the skillet you used to cook the chicken and roll it around so that the flavorful oil/butter mixture coats the corn. Grill it on a grill pan or cook it in a separate skillet until the corn is still crisp but has color on the outside. Slice off the kernels with a sharp knife and set aside.

4. To assemble the salad, pile shredded lettuce, chicken, tomatoes, cheese, corn, avocado, green onion, cilantro, and crushed chips on a big platter. Drizzle the dressing all over the top. Serve it in individual bowls.

21. Cashew Chicken Salad

Cashew Chicken Salad

Servings 2-3

Ingredients:

- 3 tablespoons low-sodium soy sauce, divided
- 2 tablespoons dry sherry
- 4 teaspoons cornstarch, divided
- 1 pound skinless, boneless chicken breast, cut into bite-sized pieces
- 1/2 cup fat-free, less-sodium chicken broth
- 2 tablespoons oyster sauce
- 1 tablespoon honey
- 2 teaspoons sesame oil, divided
- 3/4 cup chopped onion
- 1/2 cup chopped celery
- 1/2 cup chopped red bell pepper
- 1 tablespoon grated peeled fresh ginger
- 2 garlic cloves, minced

- 1/2 cup chopped green onions (about 3 green onions)
- 1/4 cup chopped unsalted dry-roasted cashews

Directions:

1. Combine 1 tablespoon soy sauce, 2 teaspoons cornstarch, and chicken in a large bowl; toss well to coat. Combine remaining 2 tablespoons soy sauce, remaining 2 teaspoons cornstarch, broth, oyster sauce, and honey in a small bowl.

2. Heat 1 teaspoon oil in a large nonstick skillet over medium-high heat. Add chicken mixture to pan; sauté 3 minutes. Remove from pan. Heat remaining 1 teaspoon oil in pan. Add onion, celery, and bell pepper to pan; sauté 2 minutes. Add ginger and garlic; sauté 1 minute. Return chicken mixture to pan; sauté 1 minute. Stir in broth mixture. Bring to a boil; cook 1 minute, stirring constantly. Remove from heat. Sprinkle with green onions and cashews.

Rice pilaf: Heat 1 tablespoon canola oil in a large saucepan over medium-high heat. Add 1/2 cup chopped onion and 2 teaspoons grated peeled fresh ginger to pan; sauté 2 minutes. Stir in 1 cup water, 1/2 cup long-grain rice, and 1/4 teaspoon salt; bring to a boil. Cover, reduce heat, and simmer 12 minutes or until liquid is absorbed. Remove from heat; stir in 2 tablespoons chopped fresh cilantro.

22. Chicken Salad Stuffed Tomatoes and Herbs

Chicken Salad Stuffed Tomatoes and Herbs
Serves 2

Ingredients:

- 6 oz. boneless skinless chicken breasts, cooked, chopped
- 1/4 cup sliced celery
- 1/4 cup chopped onions
- 3 Tbsp. Miracle Whip Light Dressing
- 1/2 tsp. dried basil leaves
- 2 medium tomatoes

Directions:

1. Combine chicken, celery and onions in medium bowl. Add combined dressing and basil; mix lightly. Cover and refrigerate at least 1 hour.

2. Cut tomatoes into wedges, starting at the top of each tomato but being careful to not cut all of the way through to bottom of tomato.

3. Place 1 tomato on each salad plate; gently separate wedges. Fill evenly with the chicken salad.

23. Warm Potato Bistro Chicken Salad

Warm Potato Bistro Chicken Salad

Servings 3

Ingredients:

- 1 lb "B" size red potatoes (about 2¼ in. in diameter)
- 1 lb chicken tenders, cut into bite-sized pieces
- 3/4 tsp salt, divided
- 1/4 tsp black pepper
- 2 tbsp white wine vinegar
- 2 tsp Dijon mustard
- 2 tsp All-Purpose Dill Seasoning Mix
- 1 tsp sugar
- 2 garlic cloves
- 3 tbsp olive oil
- 12 oz fresh green beans, trimmed and cut into 2-in. pieces
- 1 pkg torn romaine lettuce hearts (about 6 cups)

Directions:

1. Lay each potato on its side and wedge with Veggie Wedgier. In Small Batter Bowl, toss chicken with ¼ tsp of the salt and pepper.

2. Place potatoes in (12-in.) Skillet or Stir-Fry Skillet or All-Purpose Pot. Add enough cold water just to cover tops of potatoes. Cover; bring to a boil over medium heat.

3. Meanwhile, combine vinegar, mustard, seasoning mix, sugar, garlic pressed with Garlic Press, oil and remaining ½ tsp salt in Measure, Mix well.

4. When potatoes reach a boil, remove lid and place 12" Steamer onto Skillet or Pot. Add green beans to one half of Steamer and chicken to other half, spreading out slightly.

5. Cook, covered, 8-11 minutes or until chicken reaches 165°F (74°C) and green beans are crisp tender, stirring once halfway through cooking.

6. Turn off heat. Carefully lift Steamer and let water to drain into Skillet. Place Steamer on Small Easy Fit Silicone Cover to cool.

7. Drain potatoes in large Stainless Mesh Colander; cool 1-2 minutes. Place lettuce in Large Glass Mixing Bowl. Add green beans, chicken, potatoes, and dressing; toss with 3-Way Tongs. Serve warm.

24. Pistachio Cinnamon Chicken Salad with Greek Yogurt

Pistachio Cinnamon Chicken Salad with Greek Yogurt

Servings 4

Ingredients:

- 1 1/2 cups Greek yogurt
- 1/2 cup pistachios
- 1 tsp ground cinnamon
- 1 tsp fresh lime juice
- 4 fresh basil leaves
- 1 celery stalk finely chopped
- 1/4 tsp sea salt
- 1/4 tsp freshly ground pepper
- 2 scallions

Directions:

1. Shred cooked chicken breast using a fork; place in a large mixing bowl.

2. Add remaining ingredients; gently toss to combine. Transfer to serving bowls. Serve chilled or at room temperature. Sprinkle with additional scallions.

25. Garlic Sour Cream and Onion Chicken Salad

Garlic Sour Cream and Onion Chicken Salad

Servings 3-4

Ingredients:

- 2 cups shredded or diced cooked chicken
- ½ cup sour cream
- 2 tablespoons dried minced onion
- ½ teaspoon onion powder
- ¼ teaspoon garlic powder
- ¼ teaspoon salt

Directions:

1. In a medium bowl, mix all ingredients together thoroughly.
2. Serve with whole-grain crackers or fresh veggies.

3. 26. Skinny Honey Chicken Salad

Skinny Honey Chicken Salad

Servings 7

Ingredients:

- 1½ pounds boneless, skinless chicken breasts
- 2 cups low-sodium chicken broth
- 2 dried bay leaves
- ½ cup plain, non-fat Greek yogurt
- ¼ cup light mayonnaise
- 2 tablespoons apple cider vinegar
- 2 tablespoons honey
- ½ teaspoon salt
- ¼ teaspoon black pepper
- 1 cup red seedless grapes, cut in half lengthwise (20 grapes)
- ½ cup coarsely chopped unsalted, raw pecans (34 pecans)
- 1 cup diced celery (about 3 stalks)

Directions:

1. Place the chicken in a pot large enough to it all, and fill the pot with enough chicken broth to cover the chicken by about 1-2 inches. Add bay leaves, and if desired, fresh parsley stems and whole peppercorns to flavor the cooking liquid, then bring to a boil over high heat.

2. When the cooking liquid comes to a boil, cover the pot with a lid and reduce the heat to low. Simmer the chicken for 10-15 minutes, or until the internal temperature of the thickest part of the breast reaches 165°F.

3. Using tongs, remove the chicken and reserve on a plate. When it is cool enough to touch, shred it and set aside.

4. While the chicken is cooling, prepare the dressing in a large mixing bowl by whisking together the yogurt, mayonnaise, vinegar, honey, salt, and black pepper in a large mixing bowl.

5. Add the grapes, pecans, celery, and cooled chicken to the bowl, and gently toss all of the ingredients together.

6. Chill before serving.

27. Grilled Chicken Bacon and Asparagus Spinach Salad

Grilled Chicken Bacon and Asparagus
Spinach Salad

Servings 4

Ingredients:

- 1/2 pound boneless and skinless chicken breast
- salt and pepper to taste
- 1 pound asparagus, washed and trimmed
- salt and pepper to taste
- 1 tablespoon oil
- 4 strips bacon, cut into 1/2 inch pieces
- 6 cups baby spinach, washed
- 8 ounces tomatoes, diced
- 8 ounces mini bocconcini or mozzarella balls
- 1 large avocado, diced
- 1/4 balsamic vinaigrette

- 1/4 cup basil, sliced

Directions:

1. Season the chicken with salt and pepper and grill over medium-high heat until cooked, about 3-5 minutes per side before setting aside.
2. Toss the asparagus spears in the oil, salt and pepper and grill over medium-high heat until crisp-tender and slightly charred before setting aside to cool and slicing into bite sized pieces.
3. Meanwhile, cook the bacon until crispy and set aside on paper to els to drain.
4. Mix all of the ingredients and serve.

28. BONUS: 10 More Healthy Foods for Women

BONUS: 10 More Healthy Foods for Women & Nutrition Facts

1. Sweet Potatoes - Source of Vitamin A, Calcium, Vitamin C, Iron, Vitamin B6, Magnesium

2. Blueberries - Source of Vitamin A, Vitamin C, Iron, Vitamin B6, Magnesium

3. Cranberry Juice - Source of Iron, Vitamin C , Vitamin A, Magnesium, Vitamin B6

4. Green Tea - Source of Vitamin A, Vitamin C, Iron, Calcium

5. Asparagus - Source of Vitamin A, Vitamin C, Iron

6. Cod - Source of Vitamin A, Vitamin D, Calcium, Vitamin B12, Vitamin C, Iron, Vitamin B6, Magnesium

7. Bananas - Source of Vitamin A, Vitamin C , Iron, Magnesium, Vitamin B6

8. Kale - Source of Calcium, Vitamin A, Vitamin C, Magnesium, Iron, Vitamin B6, Vitamin C

9. Figs - Source of Iron, Magnesium, Vitamin C, Calcium, Vitamin A

10. Guava - Source of Vitamin C, Vitamin A, Calcium, Vitamin B6, Magnesium

29. Conclusion

Hello and thanks for downloading my book. I hope you enjoyed the recipes. My next book "Try It Now! GREEN SMOOTHIES" coming soon.

www.ingramcontent.com/pod-product-compliance
Lightning Source LLC
Chambersburg PA
CBHW060201290526
45789CB00003B/1107